THE FAST METABOLISM DIET

How to Eat More to Lose More

My 24 weeks Research and Findings with 5 overweight People on Fast Metabolism Diet

By

Jennifer Robson

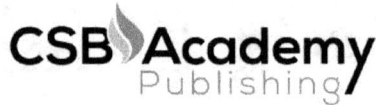

CSB Academy Publishing Company.
P. O. Box 966
Semmes, Alabama 36575, USA

Design and Layout
by
Rita Hossain
First Edition

Table of Contents

INTRODUCTION

Hey there!

If you have picked up this book for reading, chances are you are like me, finding it difficult to create a healthy balance in your life. However, I have been lucky enough to be associated with research which has led me to unearth some interesting things about some of the most popular diets out there.

This book is part of a series of three diet books and this is the last one. In my first two books, I published my research findings on "the ketogenic diet" and "the Mediterranean diet" with positive results. My profession as a freelance researcher allows me to work on a variety of projects, and when approached by a renowned company to conduct research on these diets, I found out, interestingly enough, that these are astonishingly beneficial if one needs to lose weight or/and lead a healthy life. I could not publish my findings for a period of one year, but after that had passed, I felt obliged to help other people as well through my research results.

The fact is—and this is something very personal to me— that we are leading unhealthy lives, which are contributing to health risks, obesity, diseases, and an overall lethargic lifestyle. Today, people have become comparatively more health aware and weight conscious, but there is no consensus about the diets that one can follow which are definitely going to contribute to a healthier and active lifestyle.

There are all kinds of concerns associated with diets when you come to look at it, and when you think "diet," all that comes to mind is the idea of starving yourself to near death. While that isn't the case with most diets, and most interestingly, after my research, I discovered that some of these diets are meticulously designed to trigger weight loss in our body. I have said this before in one of my previous books, and I will say it again here – our bodies are made up of a complex structure of systems which are all running smoothly and in tandem, each component being intricately tied with the rest. Careful manipulation of it can lead to weight gain or weight loss, but nowhere starvation is a solution.

A healthy weight and diet consciousness contributes to an active lifestyle. Diets work effectively when you adopt a change both internally and externally in how you conduct yourself. At least, that's what I have come to believe after the grueling research on the subject of diets and looking at some popular diets through research. In this last book, I will be discussing my research findings on the "fast metabolism diet" and how it helps lose weight. I will walk you through the concept of this diet step-by-step and will also be sharing the diet plan my research participants followed and the diet recipes. Along the way, I will clear the doubts and discuss any drawbacks associated with the diet in order to give you a complete picture of it, leaving it up to you to decide whether you would like to take up the challenge of healthy living.

I would like to add that going on a diet, as is popularly believed far from only about losing weight. It's about adopting a complete system of health consciousness where your every move and action should be calculated. You should be conscious of the meals you are consuming, the snacks you are eating, your eating habits, as well as your exercise routine. In none of the diets that I have researched on can I say that my research participants achieved positive results without some sacrifices and changes to their daily habits.

So if you want to change your life for the better and start your journey towards living healthy, you must be willing to make some sacrifices. Good things always come to those who work hard for them with patience and following any diet to be able to attain results requires a lot of patience. Results can be seen if you remain consistent.

So let's get started.

Welcome and good luck!

CHAPTER 1: EATING MORE, LOSE MORE: WHAT IS THE FAST METABOLISM DIET?

Diets like Atkins and Dukan notwithstanding with their starvation and your stomach now being unable to handle an inch more of squishy flab, you want a game changer in your life, something that will actually help you on this front. Little did you know that the tactics you previously employed with the diet plans mentioned in the beginning were not the right approach, but with *The Fast Metabolism Diet*, you will. For the diet plan is based on you **eating** – yes, you read it correctly – that will set your metabolism on fire.

Now I am sure skepticism is written all over your face already and I expect you to reluctantly skim through a few more lines to see if you can find anything to suggest I did not mean a good healthy portion of food. Unfortunately, I don't. But if you have read the other parts of this series and you instinctively trust me on this one, then I would want very much to tell you about the basics and give you a general description of what this diet is about without further ado.

What is This "Holy Grail of Weight Loss"?

It was first developed by Haylie Pomroy, also called "the metabolism whisperer," best-selling author and diet consultant to many Hollywood celebrities. Those who know her will talk about her love for food. The passion along with her profession as a food coach, as a specialized expert in diet and nutrition, prompted her to understand that rather than have an aversion to your food, count calories, and being fussy about what to eat and what not to eat, you can use it to heal your body.

According to Haylie, "[losing weight] is really not that complicated. It's not about calories or fat grams or carbs…It is about your metabolism."

At its core, therefore, you find *The Fast Metabolism Diet* stressing on boosting your metabolism with simple and practical strategies. You understand how your metabolism works, which foods can prove harmful to it. Follow the diet and for an added advantage, you effectively lose 20 pounds a month simply because it reduces insulin and hence the amount of weight you put on produced.

How is the Diet Different from Others?

Remember your expression earlier when I said you would be eating on this diet to maintain your health and figure? That's because you assume, like so many others around you, that diet equals starvation, suppressing your appetite, a limitation or lack of food or drink you consume on a regular basis, which is what the mainstream concept suggests. And in getting to the root cause of your issue, *The Fast Metabolism Diet* busts that very myth: **less food is not better**.

And rightly so, I mean the idea is not too hard to comprehend it once you think about it. You cannot get your body to burn off that extra fat if you are not providing it with the essential fuel it needs in the first place to go about it! Not just that, but once your body takes on the starvation mode, it wouldn't lose weight either now because this is the weight it deems important to survive.

This is what Haylie means with "people who always pack it in have fast metabolisms. Then there are people who hardly eat at all and remain saddled with extra weight. They are the ones with slow metabolisms that have cooled off and aren't burning the way they should."

Ready to see how it works and to kick-start your diet? Proceed to the next chapter.

CHAPTER 2: HOW DOES IT WORK?

To begin with, an understanding of how your metabolism works and why it matters as far as weight loss is concerned is important. As Haylie aptly points out, some people are naturally able to burn more calories than others are. We do have for a fact, for instance, that men burn more compared to women and that people beyond 40 years of age have to put up with a slow metabolism.

Where we may not have been able to pick our own metabolism, we can choose a diet to speed it up for you accordingly even though individuals who attempt it say it doesn't feel like 'dieting,' just simply eating healthy. In the 28-days and 3-phases of the plan, the least you can do is to understand the relationship or connection it has with your metabolism.

What is Metabolism?

Metabolism is a word we hear and use often in relation to weight loss – or weight gain– and yet we don't really know much about it except that it is the reason we could eat whatever we wanted when we were young and, ironically, now that same reason we can not lose weight. Yes, you know metabolism has something to do with your energy balance and body weight; asked what exactly and I know a few of you who will be mumbling.

 Think of your metabolism as your personal trainer working to help you burn your calories and rid your body of that fat for good. Every time that you eat, the enzymes activate to break it down and convert it into either heat, substance (muscle, blood, fat, bone), or fuel. The metabolism is involved in either storing, burning, or building. The energy, in particular, produced as a result of all these chemical processes affects everything from your mood to fertility to eating whatever you want without gaining weight; it is what keeps you alive.

So metabolism, in simpler words, can be defined as how many calories your body needs every day. The amount of time your body takes to process and burn calories from the carbs, proteins and fats you consumed is known as your metabolic rate while the amount of energy your body takes in to maintain basic functioning while you are resting is known as your basal metabolic rate.

Since you are resting at the time, it can be safe to conclude the BMR explains only 60-70% of the daily energy use; less if the individual is physically very active. The point is, it is not the only thing to determine how many calories exactly you burned within the day. It will also have to include any calorie you burned with movement or when digesting food.

Factors like your gender, age, height, weight, body makeup, certain medical disorders, climate, certain medications, and diet, a combination of which creates an imbalanced energy equation, can influence your BMR.

How do you test it?

You can get a general idea of your BMR by multiplying your weight by 10. For instance, a person who weighs 150 pounds will have a BMR of 1500 kcals. But seeing as how a number of variables/stressors such as overtraining, nutritional deficiencies, emotional and mental state, lack of sleep affect your weight loss, you may want to go ahead and check your status of metabolism with metabolic testing.

Stress and resilience spit test are recommended first to calculate your levels of certain hormones, DHEA, and cortisol. You should then measure your cardiovascular and resting metabolic (RMR) health through the Darth Vader test. The results from both these tests along with your comprehensive blood profile will signify exactly your strength and weakness.

You may not be able to control the detailed working of your metabolism, but you can control your routine, control what and how much you eat and exercise. The problem with calorie-restricted or crash diets is they reduce your BMR, forcing the body to use muscle instead for energy with a lowered muscle mass leading to a slow metabolism. This is why you gain weight so quickly once the diet ends. With *The Fast Metabolism Diet*, however, you have a plan backed by years of research and study, to ensure you eat right foods at a right time to lose weight. Let us have a closer look at this strategy.

What to Eat, What Not To Eat

The diet is basically divided into three phases, each working in coordination with the next to map out a daily menu plan that would help speed up your metabolism. The separate phases are to be recycled on a weekly basis.

Phase I – On Mondays and Tuesday (Day 1 and Day 2)

This is the stage where you consume a low-fat, moderate-protein, and a high-glycaemic diet. You are not overwhelming your body. It is just about eating foods that are easy to digest and burn, carbs being one of them. While starch and grains will be predominating your diet, your meals will constitute of proteins too; only fats remain a no-go area even for snacks. Eat carbs, including fruit, to calm down your adrenals so the body gets out from its emergency storage position.

Instructions to **unwind** include eating every 3-4 hours, five times a day. Also thrown in for good measure are physical cardio activities such as spinning or running.

Phase II – On Wednesday and Thursday (Day 3 and Day 4)

During this stage, treat yourself to a low-fat, low-carb, high-protein, and high-vegetable diet. Sounds overwhelming and difficult? It is, and perhaps the only time when you feel on a diet. But if you can bear it for these 48 hours, sticking to food like egg whites, green veggies, and deli meats, you may as well be on your way to overcoming your weight plateau.

With the body de-stressed, instructions to raise protein intake, build muscle, and **unlock** and use/burn off fat include eating every 3-4 hours, five times a day. Muscular activity, doing weights or kickboxing, also warrant a mention at this stage.

Phase III – On Friday, Saturday, and Sunday (Day 5, Day 6, and Day 7)

Given three consecutive days to use to your advantage, you are allowed to eat low-glycaemic fruits, moderate carb, moderate protein, and high healthy fat product. The idea is to not only continue burning extra fat; for the fact that it allows you to eat almost everything, it is hardly a surprise why this stage is the best part of the overall plan for most people.

Instructions to "**unleash** the burn" (heart, hormones, and heat) or speed up metabolism with the list of food having been expanded include eating five meals a day, every 3-4 hours, just like in the other 2 phases outlined. Yoga and stretching exercises come highly recommended for this phase.

What is all the uproar about calorie?

To count or to not count the calories – that is the question. And an important one too in this age. It is a good thing to see more and more people ridding themselves of the bad habits they accumulated over the years so now they can live a happier, healthier life again. But it one thing to be conscious and watchful, another to be obsessed and paranoid about it.

Having stressed that you can manipulate (with both its negative and positive connotations) your body by taking control of your metabolism, the process is further simplified by asking you NOT to count your calories when eating. As long as you are eating what and when you are told to, the 'calorie' should be of no distress to you.

How is it working?

Don't worry; we aren't delving into details regarding metabolism again. No, this is about pointing out that if in your haste you overlooked a fundamental point of value: each phase, when followed correctly, had you avoid foods, which would cause inflammation in your gastrointestinal tract. Does it matter, you ask? Yes, it does when you are trying to lose weight and the irritation just slowed down your bowels and triggered insulin resistance.

From encouraging your body to mobilizing the stored energy (in form of fat) to burning both the fat unlocked in phase 2 and the one you are eating, the following are the foods you can and cannot eat for the complete 28 days of your *Fast Metabolism Diet*:

- ✓ Fresh/cooked vegetables
- ✓ Fresh (citrus) fruits
- ✓ Beans and legumes
- ✓ Lean proteins
- ✓ Water, at least, half of your weight in ounces
- ✓ Garlic
- ✓ Green tea

- ✘ No refined sugar
- ✘ No corn
- ✘ No wheat
- ✘ No dairy
- ✘ No caffeine
- ✘ No dried fruit or fruit juice
- ✘ No alcohol
- ✘ No chemical diet or low-fat products
- ✘ No artificial sweetener
- ✘ No soy

P.S. This is not the complete list of food; you will get more ideas under Recipes. The good news, besides the apparent lack of calorie counting, is that the approved foods to satisfy your appetite with are easy to find in any grocery store and aren't exactly expensive save for some. So commitment, especially on a long-term basis, really should be no issue. Unless you are interested in knowing what is the experts' opinion about *The Fast Metabolism Diet* before you experiment it on yourself, for which I would like to direct you to the next chapter.

CHAPTER 3: DO THE EXPERTS AGREE?

Like all diets, it is alright if you are a little wary of the claims *The Fast Metabolism Diet* makes. After all, that is the only way you are going to be interested in its pros and cons, in doing your own research to see if it comes validated, and to bust associated myths instead of following it blindly. You don't mind the "challenging" part if it is worth it, right? And honestly, I wouldn't like my readers to be any less than that, so I included this section for your peace of mind.

Anyone who thinks that the new American sedentary lifestyle is becoming increasingly dependent on fast foods, which I think will be most of us willing to give up the French fries or the fizzy drinks, they would find a voice in Sarah Waybright. As a registered dietitian, she is content with how the diet shifts the focus to real whole food consumption. According to her, "Americans simply eat way too many refined, nutrient-poor carbohydrates...replacing them with nutrient-dense options like fruits, vegetables, lean protein, and fiber-rich whole grains offers a diets that's high in micronutrients for fewer calories."

She concludes by saying, "the FMD diet seems like a new way to think about an old concept: eating a diet of whole foods," which is what makes it qualitatively different from other diet programs that lack the minerals and/or vitamins offered by FMD.

Don't like how preservatives, pesticides, etc. are affecting your food? Let's see what Jasmine Jafferali, a lifestyle and wellness consultant, has to say about it. In sync with *The Fast Metabolism Diet,* she approves of Pomeroy on the point where eating organic produce is encouraged at any time possible in order to stop these elements, which when consumed worsen the liver function to burn fat. However, even as she agrees and provides her support to avoid the artificial preservatives, sugars, dyes for the ideal organic produce, she fears that such consumption may not be everyone's cup of tea either.

According to Jessica Lehmann, a registered dietitian-nutritionist, it would be excellent if people were to "learn how to plan a balanced, moderate, nutrient-dense diet that is based on a variety of whole, unprocessed foods and that fits your own individual needs and dietary preferences."

Choosing organic, while an important decision to her, doesn't mean she approves of people using "organic labeling" to defend their essentially bad food preferences. She would "much rather see someone snacking on a bowl of conventionally produced vegetables than a handful of organic cookies".

Add to it the high intake of water it recommends and you have an ecstatic Lehmann recommending it for sure, because in any case "drinking water before a meal is an easy way to fill up and reduce calorie intake."

Other professional reviewers, including Dr. Oz, have recommended it too as a "medically proven method of food as medicine to fight obesity" instead of being just another fad diet.

So, even as there are a few aspects that these professionals are not likely to recommend to their clients on the basis alone that they don't agree with those points in the first place, you do find them united on food coupled with healthy lifestyle being fundamental to a fit body.

Does that make *The Fast Metabolism Diet* okay for you? How about you preview its pros and cons yourself and decide for yourself before saying a resounding 'Yes!'?

CHAPTER 4: BENEFITS AND DRAWBACKS

First, the advantages:

- You lose about 20 pounds in a month; you will lose the extra pounds if you are overweight; if not, the diet enables you to turn into a healthier version of yourself only
- The calorie shifting concept is utilized, which is great in the sense you lose weight without reaching a plateau
- Teaches individuals the way their metabolism works, especially how some foods and eating habits can harm their metabolism
- The coordinated eating plan is meant for everyone interested in experiencing better health with the foods included; tasty recipes, clearly explained and easy-to-follow phases and tips for shopping/cooking are provided
- Organic choices are focused upon whenever possible
- Building stronger, healthier bodies is another way of saying you are boosting its ability to heal on its own
- With more energy to burn, you start leading a more active lifestyle
- Besides obesity, it minimizes risks for medical conditions like diabetes, arthritis, cardiovascular problems, celiac disease, hormonal issues, high cholesterol, infertility, and thyroid disorders
  [Note: do not take FMD as a replacement for professional medical treatment or diagnosis. Irrespective and regardless of any diagnosed medical condition, begin FMD only after you have talked to your healthcare provider first as in the case of any diet.]

Now, the disadvantages:

- It can become too restrictive at times, taking away many staple items from the diet
- It can become complicated for the individuals, a lazy dieter for instance, who aren't used to this sort of weekly rotation and switching around of fats, protein, carbs

- Exercise won't be enough to work your way out to optimal health if you are consuming a bad diet in the first place
- You can't have chocolate, caffeine, or alcohol with this diet plan
- You need to have a strict commitment to see results

At a glance, the pros seem to outweigh the cons making it such a hit with most people. The following FAQs may help you get in detail some of them, and while I wouldn't suggest any to skip it, those who are convinced already may skip these and read The Research.

1. **Is it true that there is no calorie counting when you do the fast metabolism diet?**

    Yes, it is. Given how the metabolism is not counting any, why should you? Enjoy eating the foods you love.

2. **Is it true that you have to eat *more* to lose more than the stated 20 pounds?**

    Yes, it is. You have the option to repeat the initial 28-day diet as needed until you reach (if not maintain) the desired weight goal or you may add another half-serving to what is provided for each snack or meal.

3. **Is it true that everybody benefits from the FMD lifestyle?**

    Yes, it is. This is the correct way for everyone to eat all the time. The healthy eating habits ensure you improve your mental and physical well-being regardless of the weight you need to lose; any sensitivity, allergies (e.g. dairy, wheat), or other restrictions implied by your medical condition can be worked around through the flexible plan. Your age group doesn't really matter as well; anybody following the FMD is bound to experience healthy growth and development.

    Consider vegans/vegetarians/pescetarians for instance and the meat specified in the Phases I and III. They are allowed to simply replace them with half a cup of (phase-specific) cooked legumes! Still, if you are worried about it, about getting bored, consider the fact that every phase lasts for 2-3 days, and then you can be back eating your desired food.

But just to be on the safe side, individuals who have serious medical issues, have had undergone surgery (e.g. all/part of colon removed; gastric bypass; thyroid removed), or are on hormone medications are emphasized on again about talking to their physicians before starting the diet. It is probable that your doctor divides the five meals/day option to 7-8 meals/day to make it easier for you. Not just that but the consequences of the healthy diet may even change your needs for medications, so a balance is better supervised by your doctor, right?

CHAPTER 5: THE RESEARCH

As hot as a topic metabolism is, there are a lot of myths surrounding it. In providing you the energy to shift out of bed to burning calories the whole day, the metabolism has a lot of advantages when it comes to it. Except that these often are missed, ignored, or covered up with special tricks and fad diets, which obviously do not paint the real picture across. But before you blame it for your weight gain, here's what you need to know about your metabolism and exactly how it can be tweaked for the better.

According to this study among others, which explored how sleep disorders and sleep deprivation, mounting at an alarming rate in our society, can alter our metabolism. So apart from mood and productivity, sleep-deprived individuals suffer from a reduced ability to manage their blood glucose. What's more, it's even associated with increased appetite and hunger.

Add to it the fact that a simple snack such as kale chips that too at night is encouraged by research and you have every reason not to be terrified of having to eat five times a day. Few calories, easy to digest, and packed with calcium, a basic ingredient whose deficiency leads to insomnia, makes it worth an indulgence. Similarly, if you have been keeping any feelings to hit snooze followed by skipping breakfast as you start your day, think again despite having no appetite for a quick a.m. bite. The results otherwise are not definitely not pleasant.

A step further, and we have researchers who examined how an overconsumption of low/normal/high protein would influence individual weight gain, body composition, and energy expenditure. Protein lovers rejoice! It seems as if an adequate consumption of protein equals greater energy expenditure while you guys rest.

Then again, consuming water, it has been noted, favors calorie burn during the whole day. Such a positive impact is caused by thermogenesis, i.e. your body burning calories to warm water to body temperature and regulate the whole-body metabolism. This is especially during exercise. How about you complement it and jumpstart your metabolism with quick intervals of intense exercise? Loved working out with the set of dumbbells at the local gym? One thing's for sure; you won't be letting go of them any sooner knowing that they speed up your resting metabolic rate. Or perhaps you prefer squeezing in cardio and riding a bike?

Considering a superfood? Green tea is an awesome option to be your the next-level health remedy especially when you have evidence to suggest this anti-oxidant flavored punch is not only calorie-free but also pro fast metabolism.

It's not just that we have Michelle Bridges, celebrity trainer, revealing her five superfoods as berries, kale, flax seeds, sardines, and broccoli but exclusive findings to approve you eat them in *The Fast Metabolism Diet*. A study has shown how lean beef such as chicken, turkey, fish, and beef (eaten during Phase II, often with alkalizing veggies like celery, kale, and broccoli) with its ability to reduce blood pressure can lower your chances of acquiring heart disease. That said, don't forget to top it off with a dash of cayenne pepper the next time you have a chicken or beef cooking up. Besides, if you have been questioning the intake of fat to combat fat itself since the beginning, this study might interest you, verifying that Phase III included healthy fats like avocados, olive oil, coconut, and nuts because no connection between a decline in saturated fats and the cardiovascular health was evident.

Perhaps you can see now why I believed the Americans looking to shed weight and lead a healthier life could adopt this diet. As different as it is from the one they – you – are currently living, with busy routines and fast foods overruling it, a healthy lifestyle like this one is exactly what we need. My research, therefore, was aimed to see whether it indeed is possible to stick to the plan and whether it is sustainable.

Participants

Five participants, aged 18-45, were selected for this experimental trial. The three men and two women agreed to be subject to allow us to observe the effect of diet across gender and different age groups confirm its claims.

The participants were provided with a detailed diet plan as well as the recommended exercises and their developments/problems charted for the whole period

Study

Each of the participants who signed up for the diet program was excited to see how it pans out. But we could not proceed before each of them was tested for their calorie intake to ensure that that the diet plan thus developed meticulously and provided would not be unjust to any. The following is a sample plan they were asked to follow.

	Day 1	Day 2	Day 3	Day 4	Day 5	Day 6	Day 7
Breakfast	Brown rice cereal with a big bowl of watermelon, kiwi or cantaloupe	Hot water flavored with ½ lemon squeezed along with apricot tapioca grapefruit	Egg white omelets with mushrooms, spinach, red pepper	Hot water flavored with ½ lemon squeezed along with toast with turkey bacon, jicama, and lime	Nut butter and blueberries	Fried egg and tomato with toast	Hot water flavored with ½ lemon squeezed along with sweet potato, strawberries, hashbrowns, and butter over sprouted grain toast
Snack	Pineapple smoothie	Pineapple (piece fruit)	Beef Jerky coupled with celery sticks	A mini fruit salad of apple, pear, and orange	Sweet potato chips	½ Avocado	Smoked salmon with lime, and cucumbers
Lunch	Open faced turkey sandwich	Turkey chili	Lettuce wraps along with mushroom,	Dill pickles with roast beef wrapp	Cumin beef kabobs	Spiced Turkey Burgers along with grape	1-min zucchini noodles with egg yolk, grape

			roast beef, and mushroom	ed around		tomatoes, ¼ avocado, and sweet potato chips	tomatoes, and hummus
Snack	Cherries	Pineapple	2 boiled egg whites with celery	Almond butter stuffed celery	Turkey bacon chips with guacamole	Homemade Turkey Jerky	Raw almonds and pecans
Dinner	Grilled filet mignon with steamed asparagus/broccoli and sweet potato	Vietnamese beef pho (alternating the fish sauce, soy sauce, and rice noodles with coconut amino, tamari, and brown rice pasta respectively)	Steamed white fish topped with red pepper, all-you-can-eat salad including all the veggies	Margarita pork tenderloin with asparagus	Meatballs served with spicy tomato sauce and pecans with roasted Brussels sprouts	London broil with garlic, lime, ginger marinade over arugula	Dine out

Results

The group of participants gathered at the end of every phase to provide and discuss their results. However, they were weighed at the end of every week for assessment because day-to-day fluctuations are normal, particularly after they have been on the protein-heavy Phase II; for practical reasons (read, "to avoid being discouraged for the pound gained"), they were assessed right before starting the phases over again for next week. The weight loss experienced by the five individuals is noted in the table below:

	Partipant1	Participant 2	Participant 3	Participant 4	Participant 5
Weight before diet	228	195	264	235	237
Weight after diet	176	166	198	191	189
Total weight loss	52	29	66	44	48

The shift, subtle as they are, aren't easy for everyone, especially when you have other loved ones to consider as well but the positive findings that each individual reported only encouraged them to continue with it further.

Findings and Conclusion

It's no secret that we are part of an image-conscious society where a "less-than-perfect" figure doesn't go unnoticed. The participants who agreed to follow *The Fast Metabolism Diet*, however, understood and appreciated that it wasn't only about the weight loss but about healthy eating as well. The idea of eating more was balanced with little adjustments to the diet chart to ensure each of them was equally following a strict intake pattern, which was repeated week after week for a month of dieting.

During the initial days, the men reported that they had to struggle to resist their foods like chocolate and cakes, which, rich in carbs, they would munch on as snacks for most afternoons. It was an uncontrolled over-processing of these carbohydrate items by their body, which created the fat deposits that wouldn't leave despite exercise or diet.

Where a 'normal metabolism' would have allowed you to be full and energetic for approximately four hours after eating a sandwich, an incorrect amount of insulin released at an incorrect time can usurp the optimal energy and metabolism activity your body needed leaving you craving a chocolate bar or something else that is similarly carb-loaded. But where ignoring these symptoms and not giving in was of no help to maintain your weight, a detox period followed by eating as much of the allowed foods as you want will.

The participants loved Phase I of the Diet. All of them loved fruits, and it was where they were allowed to eat most of them. That and the grains combined meant they were usually full during the phase. But in the second week, two of them noted they upped their intake of vegetables, including boiled vegetables with spices for snacks.

Other than that, each liked the fact that they could have a grain of their choice; otherwise, the large servings would have made them sick of it if they would have been asked to survive on cups of rice only. The adjustment was also made easy because the dishes were easy to prepare, particularly the snacks where a piece of fruit only was sufficient.

Exercises for Phase I was a 30 minutes session of cardio at least on both of these days. Where the male participants preferred sweating at their gym's cross trainer or bike due to their hectic work schedules, the female participants decided to perk it up to their advantage by making it a social team activity, swimming, jumping rope in their garage, or playing squash whichever was available.

Entering Phase II of the diet, any individual would typically hate it given there are only proteins to keep you company. Definitely not the most glamorous phase of all. According to the participants, this is good if you have started filling them in for your emotional cravings. If the food seems boring, you can, at least, make the most of your weight training and gym sessions this phase rewards you with. But even the meals can be tweaked a bit with your favorite herbs and spices to make them flavorsome for your attention.

Still getting hunger pangs? My participants deal with them with a big glass of water or eating more vegetables. If they were not getting enough of either, the participants stated they experienced constipation and headaches as well, although one male participant hinted his headaches might be the withdrawal symptoms of the cup of coffee he was skipping for the program. Given he was also experiencing fatigue, this seemed to be a valid factor.

As for the exercise training, improving the speed or the intensity offered them something new to focus on.

Sticking with Haylie's suggestion for doing the Phases on the exact days made things a whole lot easier as participants went from Phase II to Phase III of the diet. But again, things were easier said than done. Everyone had a tiny battle mentally where they would never think it possible they could get through the day until the results of the previous day motivated them to continue. Besides, it could be hard planning when you are allowed most foods in your diet chart.

The healthy dietary fats you receive from olive oil, raw nuts, raw seeds, or avocados are effective in triggering your body to burn stored fat only that Phase I and II set the stage for. So participants who felt it counterintuitive were encouraged to give the fat intake a try because their body had stopped losing the weight and started storing instead with the lack of dietary fat they had been eating for the past four days. The body burns through them, feels satiated, and is literally stress-free, more reason the carbs in this phase have taken a back seat. There are enough only to sustain the energy but not so much as to neglect the fat-burning process.

One participant in particular who was still finding weight loss challenging in the phase despite Phase III being such a major fat-burning period was asked to use starchy vegetables rather than grains at lunch/dinner. This way they could skip the grain for at least one day of the phase every week. Adding a multitude of fresh spices and herbs also helped support gallbladder and fat emulsification.

Add to it that you can get an appointment for a massage to have fat-burning enzymes working at your body in swelling numbers or that you can kick back cortisol levels with a couple of minutes of meditation or yoga, and this might be the best form of exercise you look forward to every week! That's not to say the participants weren't instructed not to slack on the exercise during the other two phases; a lack – or even an abundance – can truly damage your weight loss efforts.

During the weeks, there were moments when despite being provided the exact food choices they eat every day; the participants felt a little restricted by the eating plan. And they would naturally freak out or stress, which was not healthy for their body either and since it slows metabolism, it would mean all their diet efforts would be wasted.

What you have to remember at these times is that *The Fast Metabolism Diet* isn't about rapid weight loss. You would have to be wary of it if that was the case indeed because the faster it comes off, the easier it is to put back on. You may not lose as much of the pounds as you will lose the inches, especially around the hips and waist where the stubborn fat takes refuge in, without having to punish your body.

The participants said they felt happy, and well so much they wanted to keep their systems clean that way. Each of them lost weight just at different times. Each of them learned how to eat properly, from having coffee and Cheez-It's for breakfast to grain toast, eggs, or smoothie and breaking the coffee (or alcohol) addiction was the real achievement.

The best part possibly was how the diet helped their skin glow. With four weeks of eating living on organic vegetables, fruits, and nuts, the participants noted their complexion improved as the skin enjoyed natural detox and absorption of minerals and vitamins it needed to repair and rejuvenate. Even the freckles lightened up, and the hair and nails felt stronger.

They did face trouble eating out and found it hard to stick when they were at a party or at a restaurant, and the other people never understood and were offended. Not just that but participants revealed they had found the new willpower to exercise to resist all those desserts and dinner meals they were surrounded by and yet couldn't taste; two of them admitted to giving in once for their child's welcoming and at their own work anniversary respectively.

Healthy eating habits like eating breakfast and avoiding processed food were not something the 5 participants thought they would ever incorporate in their lives. But the success of the diet made them rethink their decision and so after they completed the 28-day cycle, this is what the participants remarked for their life after the experiment.

Participant 1 [Male]: He had achieved the goal weight by the end of the program and just wanted to stick to the diet simply without making a change whatsoever because he was afraid it might get him off the diet. He intended to repeat it for another month at least before reconsidering if he now feels comfortable regarding any changes to incorporate.

Participant 2 [Male]: He had achieved the goal weight too by the end of the program. Now that he was familiar with the three phases of the diet and of the specific food items that helped boost his metabolic activity, he was willing to introduce oil in multiple phases and cook healthy with it as well be it salad dressing of Phase I or full-fledged meals in Phase II or Phase III.

Participant 3 + 4 [1 Male & 1 Female]: They did not achieve the desired goal, but liked the diet enough to make it work. They were both anxious and excited about modifying the diet in a way so that it would feel like they were always eating as allowed in Phase III. The strategy was to consume only those foods that were listed for any phase. Following that, they gushed about reserving the grains for breakfast only so as to ensure they were utilized by the body or pairing desserts with the workout so as to make the activity fun and one to look out for. Another tactic under consideration was to extend Phase II, i.e. two days of Phase I would be followed by three days of Phase II and then two days of Phase III subsequently for a week or two.

Participant 5 [Female]: She completed the program successfully as well and was thinking of taking a little break before starting all over again to keep her metabolism on fire. Her work commitments require her to travel a lot, and it will be difficult to follow the plan as rigorously as she did during the experiment. During this period, however, even as she might indulge in the 'restricted' foods such as dairy, she would see that it was still the cleanest choice available like keeping it organic and free of fake sweeteners or chemicals.

If this sounds like the type of diet you can do to benefit from weight loss and a great deal of energy to leverage, then the following chapter will show you how to attempt it successfully.

CHAPTER 6: PREPARING YOURSELF FOR SUCCESS

Now that we have scientific findings to back up the theory, here comes the favorite part, I know some people have been waiting patiently since the beginning: how to go about it, how to avoid the traps others had been victim to, how to learn from their mistakes and see their efforts bore fruit.

The following dos and don'ts, expert tips, and some awesome recipes are to help you get on the scale or try the inch-tape without hesitation. This time around, you can claim you did lost weight without feeling hungry all the time or having headaches or reaching the dreaded plateau.

Dos and Don'ts

In trying to eat real food in correct portions (6 ounces of fish, 4 ounces of meat, ½-1 cup of grains) and in trying to plan your meals to keep a track of what you consume, here are what you need to implement, instructions that are key to completing each phase successfully.

- Eat five times every day or 35 times a week. Don't skip, negotiate, or compromise any snack or meal time so much so that you are to eat at the scheduled time even if you are not feeling hungry
- Eat within 30 minutes after you wake up every day. Flexibility being a positive motivator, you may prioritize and opt for a morning snack first and a breakfast later if you have to rush out within this time. This ensures you do not miss your meal, and your body has the energy it needs to function efficiently
- Eat every 3-4 hours, not counting the time you are sleeping. If you time it right, you will literally have no trouble to fit it into your schedule
- Eat foods listed for respective phase, organic whenever possible. Hold yourself accountable for not eating anything that isn't on the meal map and that includes not eating synthetic chemical products at all when possible

- Eat meat that is nitrate-free and preserved naturally and you will be on the right track to successfully completing *The Fast Metabolism Diet*
- Eat in order of the phases as outlined. In another word, you are not going to pick the phase offering foods and/or exercise of your choice; it is Phase I (2 days), then Phase II (2 days) and Phase III (3 days)
- Drink plenty of water. Do you weigh around 200 pounds? Try and drink at least 100 ounces of water daily to both flush toxins and keep yourself hydrated and satiated
- Exercise as designated for the respective phase. These have been incorporated according to and balancing the types of food included and, therefore, will work better if you follow them
- Stick to the cycle for consecutive 28 days. Honestly, after all, your attempts to be fit, you can't help but remain committed to achieving a true detox and repair of your body now, can you?
- Check with your doctor to know you are not pushing your body to another extreme while benefitting from the diet
- Set up an environment to be motivated and succeed. This includes stocking up healthy foods. And all those tempting, especially off-the-plan, foods hiding in your cupboards, pantry, and refrigerator? Allow them to take your leave and bid them a good farewell
- Minimize stress so as not to let it change your hormone profiles. A slight drop or raise and you obstruct your achievements. Now, getting plenty of sleep is one way to manage it
- Make the diet as easy as possible. In times when our comforts are dictated by how conveniently accessible they are, making meals on weekends and storing them for the whole week, shopping with plenty of time at hand to read ingredients carefully, and taking up a hobby to keep yourself distracted and the 'intense' cravings to pass helps you keep focused on the ultimate objective(s)

- Set practical goals for every week. Every time you achieve them do reward yourself with non-food items like an early bedtime or warm bath

Here is what you need to avoid

- Exercise on an empty stomach is a no-no
- Breakfast is an important meal and skipping it is definitely not encouraged particularly when you have studies suggesting that people who don't eat breakfast have more cravings or remain hungrier and, therefore, eat more during the day
- A slip is no cause to get down and not back on track with the diet plan ASAP; remember, that the most dedicated diets can slip as well
- Life may not be much 'fun' without these but given how they can be a problem and negatively influence your metabolism, dairy, soy and wheat are considered better left out in the diet – the dairy for its sugar-fat-protein ratio; the wheat for its new varieties to cause bloating, inflammation, water retention, gas, and fatigue; and the soy for its ability to mimic estrogen and contribute to belly fat

Tips

- Exploit the FMD without a gallbladder

It can be frustrating but not impossible to lose weight following the removal. How do you expect to process fats? Sure, the pancreas and liver will pitch in, but if it is a diet you are considering to take up, even if it is as healthy as *The Fast Metabolism Diet* is, what helps?

For one, slowing down and chewing the food well does. Like approx. 40 times for every mouthful. Second, you can be willing for loading up on fresh herbs and spices. Take basil, fennel, turmeric, cilantro or dried spices like ginger, hot peppers, hot paprika, cayenne, and you literally lighten the load your pancreas/liver receives. For the foods themselves, options like lima beans, bigger veggies including asparagus and kale, fresh figs, cucumbers, sweet potatoes, lemons, tomatoes are always preferable. Digestive bitters before every meal is another good idea to improve your digestion.

- Know which dietary supplements to avoid throughout the diet

Certain supplements can be taken with the FMD but noting that the Phase I and II are strict on restricting the intake of fats and oils, you need to make sure your supplements don't constitute such ingredients during the respective stages. That said, check with the health care practitioner before continuing supplementation with the FMD.

- Keep yourself from feeling deprived

That would have been a difficult one to answer for any other diet. Except for a few selected items, the flexibility is such that you can enjoy your meals to the fullest. And if it is the servings that bother you, you always change the dishes – use smaller plates instead – to modify and relish an impression that you are eating more food.

Consider yourself ready to go, keep the stress down and your diet up by not leaving the house without water and a phase-appropriate snack. As strange as it sounds, it would probably take you some time to getting used to drinking all that water because the majority of Americans are supposed to be chronically dehydrated. Keep a water bottle in your car to sip at every signal, for instance. If drinking water seems boring, use mint leaves and a lime wedge to add natural flavor.

- Cook for the entire family

Like any other homemade meals you enjoy with your loved ones, you can ensure there are no complaints in this regard as well if, for instance, besides going generic, you take the word "diet" out of it. Like your reaction, in the beginning, it's natural that your loved ones are thinking along the same way too: that diet equals not just unpalatable food but of skimpy portions as well. Take a look at the super-quick and phase-appropriate meals I have included in the next section and tell me if it's not 'regular' eating. And if it's a conscious choice they are making to avoid the fast metabolism lifestyle, don't stop them from adding sour cream, cheese, flour tortilla or hamburger bun as suitable for the dish and their respective taste.

For the one responsible for all that cooking – there will a lot of it mind you – it's practical to cook extra and freeze the leftovers. It is also smart if you began by writing an inventory log for each phase, so you don't lose track of the meals already frozen.

- Understand your body

This is often the most understated tip offered regarding *The Fast Metabolism Diet*. For the time both before you start on the diet and as you progress on it, you have to have an understanding of how your body works with respect to food and eating. The consequence of not doing it means you are going to remain stressed, confused, or depressed over your health and body. So, does that mean a major in Anatomy is in order? Of course not! But a general know-how of which foods and how much of it, you and your body can process without any issue. And while you are at it, make peace with your food so (for once) you may actually look forward to eating all your favorite foods.

Chapter 7: RECIPES

Please note that the nutritional information of the following recipes may differ according to your ingredients. The ones provided are therefore to be used as reference only.

Blueberry Zucchini Smoothie

Phase 3, this refreshing recipe serves 1

Ingredients:

- 1 small zucchini, peeled if not organic
- A handful of spinach
- ½ banana
- 1 cup blueberries
- 1 cup coconut water
- ½ cup water
- 1-2 dates or 5-8 drops of liquid stevia
- ½ tbsp chia seeds

For topping

- 1 tbsp wild blueberries
- 1 tbsp almond butter

Preparation Method:

1. Put all the ingredients in a blender or a smoothie maker and blend on high until smooth.
2. Pour it out and top it with wild blueberries and almond butter before serving.

Nutritional Information: 236 calories; 4g fat; 51g carbohydrates; 5g protein.

Chicken and Barley Soup

Phase I, this delicious recipe serves 6

Ingredients:

- 2 ½ lbs boneless, skinless chicken breast
- 4 cups vegetable broth
- 4 cups chicken broth
- 2 cups water
- 1 cup diced onion
- 1 whole bay leaf
- 1 tbsp minced garlic
- 2 cups cubed and peeled butternut squash
- 1 whole bay leaf
- 2 cups cubed yellow summer squash
- ¼ tsp sea salt
- 2 cups cubed zucchini squash
- ¼ tsp black pepper
- 1 cup chopped broccoli florets
- 1 cup barley
- 8 oz chopped fresh mushrooms

Preparation Method:

1. Pour in the broth and water into a large soup pan.
2. Add in chicken, garlic, onion, salt, bay leaf, pepper. Get it to a boil.
3. Then cook low for 1 hour. Add barley and veggies to soup pot.
4. Bring to boil and then simmer on low further for an hour or two until you see the veggies taking the desired textured form.
5. Serve it hot.

Nutritional Information: 433.3 calories; 7.7g fat; 44.0g carbohydrates; 48.7g protein.

Spanish Egg White Scramble

Phase II, this delectable recipe serves 1

Ingredients:

- 3 egg whites
- 1 tbsp chopped shallot
- 1 tbsp chopped onion
- 1 tbsp minced green chili pepper
- 1 tbsp minced garlic
- ¼ tsp crushed red pepper flakes
- ¼ tsp dried parsley/cilantro or 1tsp fresh
- ½ c. chopped fresh spinach
- Sea salt to taste

Preparation Method:

1. Heat 1tsp water in a nonstick pan and cook shallot, onion, green chilies, and garlic until they turn soft.
2. Add in spinach. Cook until it is wilted.
3. Add eggs. Scramble together and add the rest of the ingredients. Platter it out.

Nutritional Information: 108.0 calories; 0.2g fat; 10.1g carbohydrates; 16.6g protein.

Steak and Asparagus Lettuce Wraps

Phase II, this scrumptious recipe serves 2

Ingredients:

- 8 asparagus spears
- 10 oz. round steak in strips
- ½ tsp minced garlic
- ½ lime, juiced

- ½ tsp dried cilantro
- 4 leaves, romaine
- ¼ tsp red pepper flakes, crushed
- Balsamic vinegar/mustard to taste
- Salt and pepper to taste

Preparation Method:

1. Preheat your broiler and then place it in the oven.
2. Put in the asparagus and steak into a foil pouch.
3. Whisk the garlic, salt, red pepper flakes pepper, cilantro, and lime juice together in a small bowl. Drizzle it over the asparagus and steak.
4. Seal the pouch, put in on the broiler pan. Leave it to broil for 25 minutes; alternatively, until the steak is done.
5. Take out the pouch. Let the steam vent from one end only.
6. Then pour the liquid from the pouch into a small bowl and mix it with some vinegar/mustard.
7. Start dressing up your plate with a lettuce leaf on each. Spoon half the asparagus and steak mixture on each leaf. Place another lettuce leaf on top of it, roll, and eat.

Nutritional Information: 206.7 calories; 5.7g fat; 4.0g carbohydrates; 34.2g protein.

Green Apple, Spinach, and Tuna Salad

Phase I, this mouth-watering recipe serves 2

Ingredients:

- 1 c. chopped apple
- 2 c. spinach
- 5 oz can solid white tuna (in water)
- ½ c. peeled, diced cucumber
- 1 tbsp minced red onion
- ½ c. diced carrot

- ½ lemon or balsamic

Preparation Method:

1. Drain the tuna and place it in a bowl.
2. Add all the ingredients. Stir well.

Nutritional Information: 164.7 calories; 1.2g fat; 25.5g carbohydrates; 15.8g protein.

Salad Dressing and Veggie Dip

Phase II, this yummy recipe serves 6

Ingredients:

- 1 tsp dill
- 2 tsp parsley/cilantro
- 1 tbsp apple cider vinegar/balsamic
- ½ c. chopped, peeled cucumber
- ½ Truvia or stevia
- 1 chopped garlic clove
- Sea salt to taste

Preparation Method:

1. Place all your ingredients into a blender. Blend until it's smooth.

Nutritional Information: 3.4 calories; 0.0g fat; 0.7g carbohydrates; 0.1g protein.

Coconut Curry Chicken

Phase III, this wonderful recipe serves 4

Ingredients:

- 1 lb. skinless, boneless, chopped chicken breast
- 14 oz. can coconut milk

- ½ c. cooked quinoa
- 1 c. canned, diced tomatoes
- 3 c. spinach
- 1 tbsp olive oil
- 2 tbsp tomato paste
- 1 med. chopped onion
- 2 tsp curry powder
- 1 tsp sea salt

Preparation Method:

2. Heat the oil in a skillet.
3. Add salt and onion. Sauté for approximately 7 minutes or until soft.
4. Add curry powder. Sauté again until you see that the onions are coated.
5. Add tomatoes, tomato paste, coconut milk. Stir occasionally for nearly 5 minutes until the mixture starts to thicken.
6. Put in the chicken. Cook until it is cooked thoroughly.
7. Add in spinach; stir until wilted.
8. Serve over quinoa.

Nutritional Information: 277.6 calories; 11.2g fat; 15.5g carbohydrates; 28.8g protein.

Open-Faced Turkey Sandwich

Phase I, this favorite recipe serves 1

Ingredients:

- 2 oz. turkey or chicken deli meat
- 1 plum, sliced tomato
- 1 slice sprouted grain bread
- Large romaine lettuce leaf
- 1 tbsp mustard
- Slice of onion

- Pepper to taste
- Sea salt to taste

Preparation Method:

1. Spread a layer of mustard on the bread.
2. Place the rest on top.
3. Sprinkle salt and pepper to season it. Ready to serve.

Nutritional Information: 168.8 calories; 1.8g fat; 23.6g carbohydrates; 14.7g protein.

Rosemary Pork Roast (with Sweet Potato)

Phase I, this nutritional recipe serves 8

Ingredients:

- 2 tbsp olive oil
- 2 lbs boneless pork loin
- ½ tsp dried rosemary
- ½ tsp black pepper
- ½ tsp dried thyme
- ½ tbsp sea salt
- ½ dried sage
- 6 garlic cloves

Tips

Peeling and cutting 4 large or 8 small sweet potatoes to add on top of the pork in the slow cooker.

Preparation Method:

1. Keep aside the garlic and pork while mixing the rest of the ingredients together.
2. Rub the mixture thoroughly on the meat.
3. Make small marks in meat and stick the garlic down by its side.

4. Place it in the slow cooker. Make sure it's set on low before you leave it for 8-10 hrs; set it at 'high' if you are thinking of cooking 6-8 hrs.

Nutritional Information: 219.8 calories; 9.0g fat; 0.9g carbohydrates; 32.1g protein.

Chicken Sausage with Brown Rice Fusilli

Phase I, this excellent recipe serves 4

Ingredients:

- 12 oz. chicken/turkey sausage
- 2 c. cooked brown rice fusilli or another type
- 1 tbsp crushed garlic
- 1 c. chopped broccoli florets
- 2 c. cubed zucchini
- ¼ c. minced red onion
- Sea salt to taste
- Pepper to taste

Preparation Method:

1. Begin by preparing the pasta as per the directions on the box.
2. When done, strain and rinse it out.
3. Preheat nonstick skillet.
4. Cut the sausage into pieces then add these pieces along with garlic, onion, and 1-2 tbsp of water. Keep it at medium heat and cook until slightly brown.
5. Throw in the remaining ingredients. Let it be until the veggies are completely cooked.
6. Add in pasta. Wait until it is warm before serving.

Nutritional Information: 588.7 calories; 6.1g fat; 91.4g carbohydrates; 30.4g protein.

Oatmeal with Blueberries and Cinnamon

Phase III, this thrilling recipe serves 1

Ingredients:

- ½ fresh or frozen blueberries
- ½ c. cooked steel-cut oats
- ¼ c. sunflower seeds/walnuts/pecans/etc
- Ground cinnamon to taste
- Stevia to taste

Preparation Method:

1. Cook your oats as per the directions. Or let them soak overnight in 1 c. Water and then simmer oats and water in a saucepan the next morning for nearly 30 minutes.
2. When cooked, top them with the remaining ingredients to serve and enjoy.

Nutritional Information: 375.8 calories; 18.9g fat; 44.1g carbohydrates; 11.5g protein.

Avocado Quesadilla

Phase III, this highly rated recipe serves 1

Ingredients:

- ½ smashed avocado
- 1 sprouted grain tortilla
- ½ tsp basil
- ½ tsp dried rosemary
- ½ tsp oregano
- ½ tsp grapeseed oil
- ¼ lime juice
- Sea salt to taste

- ¼ tsp safflower mayo

Preparation Method:

1. Heat the oven to 350 deg.
2. Brush the tortilla lightly with oil. Sprinkle herbs and salt and bake it for 10 minutes.
3. During that time, combine the mayo, avocado, and lime juice.
4. Take out a tortilla and spread the avocado mixture on top to serve.

Nutritional Information: 279.1 calories; 7.1g fat; 25.4g carbohydrates; 2.1g protein.

Additional Recipes

For a bonus, here are more recipes for you to try your skills at

Watermelon Pizza

Phase I, this one-of-a-kind recipe serves 1

Ingredients:

- 1 watermelon slice with its rind removed and almost an inch thick
- 2 tbsp water
- 2 tbsp unseasoned rice vinegar
- ½ medium-size red onion, thin sliced
- 1 tbsp fresh lemon juice
- ¼ tsp sea salt
- 2 tsp nutritional yeast
- ½ cup organic canned garbanzo beans
- 1 ½ cups organic mixed baby greens
- 5 drops liquid stevia

Dressing:

- 1 tbsp unseasoned rice vinegar
- 1 tbsp fresh lemon juice

- 1 tsp Dijon mustard
- 1 tsp grain mustard
- 1/8 tsp sea salt
- 6 drops liquid stevia

Preparation Method:

1. In a small bowl, add sliced onion, unseasoned rice vinegar, water, sea salt, lemon juice, and liquid stevia and toss them well. Keep it aside to marinate for 10 minutes.
2. For the dressing, mix all the ingredients well. Refrigerate until you are ready to use it.
3. Discard the liquid of the marinated onions and add them to the mixed greens and garbanzo beans in a salad bowl. Pour over half of the dressing; add more to suit your taste. Toss well.
4. Now, place the watermelon on a plate and arrange this salad on top of it to create a 'pizza' look. Sprinkle nutritional yeast above it. Serve with any Phase I grain.

Carrot-Oat Breakfast Cookies

Phase III, this creative recipe makes 12 cookies

Ingredients:

- 1 cup rolled oats
- ¾ cup chopped walnuts
- ¾ cup grated carrot
- ¾ cup baking mix
- ½ cup xylitol
- ¼ cup coconut or almond milk
- 1 egg
- 1 ½ tsp cinnamon
- 1 ½ tsp baking powder
- 1 tbsp melted coconut oil

Preparation Method:

1. Preheat your oven to 375°F.
2. Put all the dry ingredients together in a bowl and whisk them.
3. Take another bowl and beat the egg in it. Pour in oil and milk. Add carrots.
4. Add the wet mixture to the dry ingredients and stir together to combine. Throw in the walnuts.
5. Scoop out 12 cookies onto a parchment-lined baking sheet. Bake for 12-15 minutes or until you see their bottoms become a light brown.

Detox Smoothie

Phase II, this easy-to-make recipe serves 2

Ingredients:

- ½ cup peeled and diced cucumbers
- ½ cup coarsely chopped kale with its ribs removed
- ½ tsp minced ginger
- ½ tsp fresh and chopped parsley
- 1 tbsp spirulina
- 1 cup ice cubes

Preparation Method:

1. Put all the ingredients into a blender along with 2 cups of water. Blend until smooth. Serve right away.

Rhubarb Mousse

Phase II, this food lover's recipe serves 6

Ingredients:

- 2 large, fresh egg whites
- 1 cup xylitol
- 4 cups of fresh rhubarb in 1/2 –inch pieces
- 1/8 tsp cream of tartar

- ¼ tsp cinnamon
- 1 tsp vanilla
- 2 tbsp lemon juice

Preparation Method:

2. Put lemon juice, rhubarb, cinnamon, and xylitol into a large saucepan.
3. Stir to combine them over medium heat. Do this until the xylitol has completely dissolved. Then bring the pan's heat to medium-low, cover it and let it simmer for approximately 7 minutes or until the rhubarb is tender. You can stir occasionally.
4. Pour in the vanilla. Let the mixture cool at room temperature.
5. Take an electric mixer and beat the egg whites and the cream of tartar together until you see a stiff peak forming.
6. Stir ¼ of this egg white with the now-cooled rhubarb mixture. Gently fold in the remaining mixture.
7. Scoop into individual dishes and let it chill before serving.

CHAPTER 8: MY FINAL THOUGHTS

Most of us remain unaware of the secret weight that our bodies are taking in until we no longer can fit into our favorite dresses. And like all things serious, the realization opens a Pandora box and everything seems to go haywire. You have a special event to attend around the corner, you can't give up the few precious minutes of beauty sleep in the morning within a tight schedule for a walk, and then with the stress ultimately getting to you, you start craving all sorts of crazy stuff even if you have been a careful eater before.

The Metabolism Diet claims to help one lose 20 pounds in 28 days. Leaving the *fad not fad* debate behind, here is a solution that promises to do something about your problems before everything gets out of your hand. You knew dieting, and clean eating would call for a discipline. But I know how shedding weight and eating organic foods are not just attractive enough as advantages to joining fellow dieters.

As my research showed, making better food choices and drinking lots of water not only reset the metabolism and kept the weight off but also improved their overall look, so they stopped feeling crap every time they looked into the mirror. The dull and dry skin had been replaced flawlessly as day after day they ate lean proteins, fresh fruit, whole grains, organic veggies, and drank a good quantity of lemon water.

There is no calorie counting. The whole 'diet' is about understanding how your body has been designed to work and establishing that it does function that way. Processed and fast foods makeup only a fraction of the pollution and stress you experience in daily life, which is why eating clean food in set proportions distributed through the day is coupled with simple yet effective exercise for optimal efficiency. And the phases – they are simply a strategic and systematic rotation of the nutritious foods to facilitate body transformation as it switches between the active recovery and rest stages of its metabolism.

Anyone who is not determined to improve their relationship with the food they eat and their own body first is, according to Haylie, not suitable for this diet. The results from my research work do not disown this idea. While the five individuals did agree to be part of the study, the follow-ups clearly showed that had it not been a scientific observation, their routines and habits would have possibly allowed for more slip-ups than they currently experienced.

The faint of the heart will always have excuses at the ready: organic stuff is more expensive than they can afford; they do not find it tasty; it takes a lot of effort to prepare new dishes; the diet means you are spending more time in the kitchen than in any other room; etc. And that's just the list for the food; exercises are entitled to one of their own.

Now these objections can be true if you want, or you can try and be a smart shopper, planning your meals in advance according to the ingredients available easily, cooking them up and freezing them for later. The diet challenges you not to give excuses to eat real food, to hydrate properly, to start lifting weight or getting soothing massages. Any phase that you think looks complicated, you can carefully plan it over the week so that it can be 'enjoyed' over the weekend only and you won't feel exhausted. You see, the diet will even support your daily routine in some instances as long as you drink plenty of water; feed your body well; are kind to your body (e.g. breathing, spa treatments are so integral to manage your body); and move and exercise.

This is exactly what interested me the most and what I wanted to share with all of you out there. The research produced all the evidence already on the subject, and I did some on my own before recommending it to you. And it's not just about the 28 days. It can easily be worked into a lifelong effort; you can go on to lose 70 or more pounds and not quit. Just do ask your healthcare provider to see it is alright for you, especially for individuals taking supplements or recovering from any illness or surgery.

If long-term well being is your goal, then I suggest you simply repeat the nutrient-dense foods as illustrated in these phases, but instead of letting your body adapt or you getting bored with it, keep it interesting by bringing in variety like trying new foods, new sports, new recipes, or add holistic health practices in your everyday life. Maintain a journal as you notice the way your body is responding to the diet plan so you may alter and customize it accordingly. Also, while I did gave you a good base to build upon, it would be great if you could take some time out and read up on how your body works and how this diet works for it. When you know what is important, you can strive for more improvements. And that is what I wish you best of luck with, not just the initial month but for a lifetime of enjoying *The Fast Metabolism Diet.*

Lastly, as I mentioned before my background is in research and not book writing, so please forgive me for any errors or typos I may have made here. Also, a humble request, if you think I was able to help you any, please give me a good review on Amazon where I will be publishing this book.

Thank you for reading and good luck with your journey into a great health and long life.